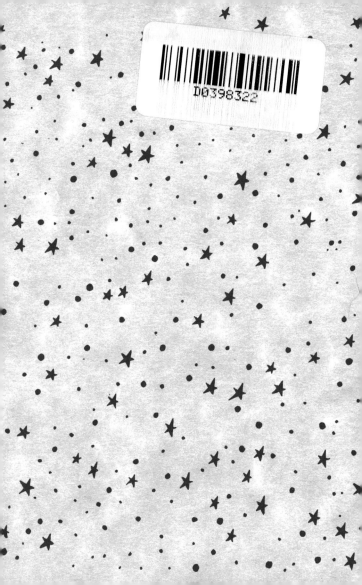

A Dancing Star

A Dancing Star

Inspirations to Guide and Heal

Edited by
Eileen Campbell

The Aquarian Press
An Imprint of HarperCollins*Publishers*

The Aquarian Press
An Imprint of GraftonBooks
A Division of HarperCollins*Publishers*
77–85 Fulham Palace Road,
Hammersmith, London W6 8JB

Published by The Aquarian Press 1991
1 3 5 7 9 10 8 6 4 2

A CIP record for this book
is available from the British Library

IBN 1-85538-101-X

Typeset by Harper Phototypesetters Limited,
Northampton, England
Printed by HarperCollinsManufacturing,
Hong Kong

I say to you: 'One must have chaos in oneself in order to give birth to a dancing star.'

FRIEDRICH NIETZSCHE

Introduction

The Nietzsche quote from which this anthology takes its title illustrates the exciting potentiality of the dancing star emerging from chaos.

Our lives are constantly subject to change, and frequently chaos ensues, both within and without. Dreams, relationships, plans seldom work out as we had hoped; disappointment, failure, illness, and finally death itself, cannot be avoided. Suffering is part of the human condition, but our problems are never as unique as we feel them to be. Throughout history others have trod the same path of human experience and have had insight into how we can rise above the circumstances we find ourselves in.

At times we all need inspiration — to make a major change in our lives, to help us deal with some unexpected, and perhaps tragic, life event, to comfort us when we feel we have lost our way and life has lost its meaning.

Invariably chaos in our lives brings transformation in its wake. Here lies our greatest opportunity to learn and grow. With inspiration comes the necessary shift of consciousness — and healing.

This anthology of quotations is gathered from both

East and West, from the great spiritual teachers of all religious traditions and from philosophers and psychologists, playwrights, novelists and poets of both the past and the present.

It has been a wonderfully rewarding experience for me to gather these quotations together. I hope that the selection will prove as inspiring and helpful to others as it has been for myself.

The words that enlighten the soul are more precious than jewels.

HAZRAT INAYAT KHAN

Go confidently in the direction of your dreams! Live the life you've imagined.

As you simplify your life, the laws of the universe will be simpler; solitude will not be solitude, poverty will not be poverty, nor weakness weakness.

HENRY DAVID THOREAU

Lord, we know what we are, but know not what we may be.

WILLIAM SHAKESPEARE
Hamlet IV.

There is no coming to consciousness without pain.

C.G. JUNG

Truly, it is in the darkness that one finds the light, so when we are in sorrow, then this light is nearest of all to us.

MEISTER ECKHART

*Be willing to accept the shadows
that walk across the sun*

*If this world were a perfect place
where would souls go to school*

*Do not weep for the limitations
that you see existing in your world.
Those limitations are there for a purpose.*

*Where would there be an opportunity to
  learn
if not in the world of imperfection?*

*Do not grieve for those who suffer,
who are subjected to limited capacities for
  living.*

*View your world as a transient place
where souls choose to come*

because this is what they have selected
as their mode of learning
to the most minute detail.

EMMANUEL

Weeping may endure for a night, but joy cometh in the morning.

Psalm 30:5

Life is not the way it's supposed to be.
It's the way it is. The way you cope
with it is what makes the difference.

VIRGINIA SATIR

Change cannot be avoided . . . Change provides the opportunity for innovation. It gives you the chance to demonstrate your creativity.

KESHAVAN NAIR

Do not weep; do not wax indignant.
Understand.

BARUCH SPINOZA

In this evanescent panorama of life all things and objects are subject to transmutation and dissolution. The Lord alone is real, with whom we are eternally united.

SWAMI RAMDAS

Behold but One in all things; it is the second that leads you astray.

KABIR

False imagination teaches that such things as light and shade, long and short, black and white are different and are to be discriminated; but they are not independent of each other; they are only different aspects of the same thing, they are terms of relation, not of reality. Conditions of existence are not of a mutually exclusive character; in essence things are not two but one.

Lankavatara Sutra

One in All,
All in One —
If only this is realized,
No more worry about your not being
     perfect!

SENG-TS'AN

Do not take life's experiences too seriously. Above all, do not let them hurt you, for in reality they are nothing but dream experiences . . .

If circumstances are bad and you have to bear them, do not make them a part of yourself.

Play your part in life, but never forget that it is only a role.

PARAMAHANSA YOGANANDA

Even a happy life cannot be without a measure of darkness and the word 'happiness' would lose its meaning if it were not balanced by sadness.

C.G. JUNG

Life can only be understood backwards;
it has to be lived forwards.

SØREN KIERKEGAARD

One day a man of the people said to Zen Master Ikkyu: 'Master, will you please write for me some maxims of the highest wisdom?' Ikkyu immediately took his brush and wrote the word 'Attention.' 'Is that all?' asked the man. 'Will you not add something more?' Ikkyu then wrote twice running: 'Attention. Attention.' 'Well,' remarked the man rather irritably, 'I really don't see much depth or subtlety in what you have just written.' Then Ikkyu wrote the same word three times running: 'Attention. Attention. Attention.' Half-angered, the man demanded: 'What does that word 'attention' mean anyway?' And Ikkyu answered gently: 'Attention means attention.'

PHILIP KAPLEAU

As a man thinks, so does he become.
Every man is the son of his own works.

CERVANTES

*Every thought you have
makes up some segment
of the world you see.
It is with your thoughts, then,
that we must work,
if your perception of the world
is to be changed.*

A Course in Miracles

If a man lives without inner struggle, if everything happens in him without opposition . . . he will remain such as he is.

G.I. GURDJIEFF

The truth is that life is hard and dangerous; that he who seeks his own happiness does not find it; that he who is weak must suffer; that he who demands love, will be disappointed; that he who is greedy, will not be fed; that he who seeks peace, will find strife; that truth is only for the brave; that joy is only for him who does not fear to be alone; that life is only for the one who is not afraid to die.

JOYCE CAREY

It is not because things are difficult that we do not dare; it is because we do not dare that they are difficult.

SENECA

The human condition is such that pain and effort are not just symptoms which can be removed without changing life itself; they are rather the modes in which life itself, together with the necessity to which it is bound, makes itself felt. For mortals, the 'easy life of the gods' would be a lifeless life.

HANNAH ARENDT

What doesn't kill me, makes me stronger.

ALBERT CAMUS

The life of man on earth, my lord, in comparison with the vast stretches of time about which we know nothing, seems to me to resemble the flight of a sparrow, who enters through a window in the great hall warmed by a blazing fire laid in the centre of it, where you feast with your councillors and liegemen, while outside the tempests and snows of winter rage. And the bird swiftly sweeps through the great hall and goes out the other side, and after this brief respite from winter, he goes back into winter and is lost to your eyes. Such is the brief life of man, of which we know neither what goes before nor what comes after . . .

VENERABLE BEDE

No one knows whether death may not turn out to be the greatest of blessings for a human being; and yet people fear it as if they knew for certain that it is the greatest of evils.

SOCRATES

All birth ends in death.
All creation ends in dissolution.
All accumulation ends in dispersion.
All that appears real is transitory.
. . . Come,
Drink the elixir of fearlessness!

NAGARJUNA

With courage you will dare to take risks, have the strength to be compassionate and the wisdom to be humble. Courage is the foundation of integrity.

KESHAVAN NAIR

*Most people think that external life will give them what they crave and seek . . . Life comes in as impressions and it is here that it is possible to **work on oneself** . . . No one can transform external life. But everyone can transform his impressions.*

MAURICE NICOLL

What we vividly imagine, ardently desire, enthusiastically act upon, must inevitably come to pass.

COLIN P. SISSON

When one door closes another opens.
Expect that new door to reveal even
greater wonders and glories and
surprises. Feel yourself grow with
every experience. And look for the
reason for it.

EILEEN CADDY

People travel to wonder at the height of mountains, at the huge waves of the sea, at the long courses of rivers, at the vast compass of the ocean, at the circular motion of the stars; and they pass by themselves without wondering.

ST AUGUSTINE

He who would know the world, seek first within his being's depths; he who would truly know himself, develop interest in the world.

RUDOLF STEINER

Man, enter into thyself. For this
*   Philosophers' Stone*
Is not to be found in foreign lands.

ANGELUS SILESIUS

Teach me my God and King
In all things thee to see
And what I do in anything
To do it as for thee.

A servant with this clause
Makes drudgerie divine
Who sweeps a room as for thy laws
Makes that and the action fine.

This is the famous stone
That turneth all to gold;
For that which God doth touch and own
Cannot for less be told.

GEORGE HERBERT

A human being is part of the whole,
called by us 'Universe'; a part limited in
time and space. He experiencies himself,
his thoughts, and feelings as something
separated from the rest — a kind of
optical delusion of his consciousness.
This delusion is a kind of prison for
us, restricting us to our personal desires
and to affection for a few persons nearest
to us.

Our task must be to free ourselves
from this prison by widening our circle of
compassion to embrace all living
creatures, and the whole of nature in its
beauty.

ALBERT EINSTEIN

Things of a day! What are we, and what are we not? A dream about a shadow is man: yet, when some god-given splendour falls, a glory of light comes over him and his life is sweet.

PINDAR

People are like stained-glass windows. They sparkle and shine when the sun is out, but when the darkness sets in, their true beauty is revealed only if there is a light from within.

ELISABETH KÜBLER-ROSS

There can be no Kingdom of God in the world without the Kingdom of God in our hearts.

ALBERT SWEITZER

Let there be many windows in your soul
That all the glory of the universe
May beautify it. Not the narrow pane
Of one poor creed can catch the radiant rays
That shine from countless sources. Tear
    away
The blinds of superstition; let the light
Pour through fair windows broad as
    truth itself
And high as Heaven.
Why should the spirit peer
Through some priest-curtained orifice,
    and grope
Along dim corridors of doubt, when all
The splendour from unfathomed seas of
    space
Might bathe it with their golden seas of
    love?
Sweep up the debris of decaying faiths,

Sweep down the cobwebs of worn-out
    beliefs,
And throw your soul wide open to the light
Of reason and of knowledge. Tune your ear
To all the wordless music of the stars,
And to the voice of nature, and your heart
Shall turn to truth and goodness, as the
    plant
Turns to the sun. A thousand unseen
    hands
Reach down to help you from their
    peace-crowned heights,
And all the forces of the firmament
Shall fortify your strength. Be not afraid
To thrust aside half-truths and grasp the
    whole.

RALPH WALDO TRINE

In every corner of my soul, there is an altar to a different god.

FERNANDO PESSOA

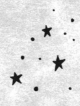

　　　　　. . . And I have felt
A presence that disturbs me with the joy
Of elevated thoughts; a sense sublime
Of something far more deeply interfused,
Whose dwelling is the light of setting
　　suns,
And the round ocean and the living air,
And the blue sky, and in the mind of
　　man:
A motion and a spirit, that impels
All thinking things, all objects of all
　　thought,
And rolls through all things.

WILLIAM WORDSWORTH

True joy is not an emotional state. It is not that which one feels when some desire is satisfied, or when everything at last goes well. It is inward; it is of the soul.

J. DONALD WALTERS

Who looks outside dreams; who looks inside wakes.

C.G. JUNG

The morning glory which blooms
for an hour
Differs not at heart from the giant pine,
Which lives for a thousand years.

Zen poem

The Tao gives birth to all beings,
nourishes them, maintains them,
cares for them, comforts them, protects
    them,
takes them back to itself,
creating without possessing,
acting without expecting
guiding without interfering.
That is why love of the Tao
is in the very nature of things.

LAO-TZU

More things are wrought by prayer
Than this world dreams of.

ALFRED TENNYSON

We do not understand that life is paradise, for it suffices only to wish to understand it, and at once paradise will appear in front of us in its beauty.

FYODOR DOSTOYEVSKY

Though I speak with the tongues of men and of angels, and have not charity, I am become as sounding brass, or a tinkling cymbal.

And though I have the gift of prophecy, and understand all mysteries, and all knowledge; and though I have all faith, so that I could remove mountains, and have not charity, I am nothing.

And though I bestow all my goods to feed the poor, and though I give my body to be burned, and have not charity, it profiteth me nothing.

Charity suffereth long, and it is kind; charity envieth not; charity vaunteth not itself, is not puffed up.

Doth not behave itself unseemly, seeketh
not her own, is not easily provoked,
thinketh no evil;

Rejoiceth not in iniquity, but rejoiceth
in the truth;

Beareth all things, believeth all things,
hopeth all things, endureth all things.

Charity never faileth . . .

1 Corinthians 13:1–8

Love gives naught but itself and
takes naught but from itself.
Love possesses not nor would it
be possessed;
For love is sufficient unto love.

KHALIL GIBRAN

One never loves enough.

ALDOUS HUXLEY

There is hunger for ordinary bread, and there is hunger for love, for kindness, for thoughtfulness, and this is the great poverty that makes people suffer so much.

MOTHER TERESA

*Sell your cleverness and buy
bewilderment.*

JALAL-UDDIN RUMI

A man can only do what he can do.
But if he does that each day he can sleep
at night and do it again the next day.

ALBERT SCHWEITZER

To laugh often and love much, to win
the respect of intelligent persons and the
affection of children; to earn the
approbation of honest critics and to
endure the betrayal of false friends; to
appreciate beauty; to find the best in
others; to give one's self; to leave the
world a bit better, whether by a healthy
child, a garden patch or a redeemed
social condition; to have played and
laughed with enthusiasm and sung with
exultation; to know even one life has
breathed easier because you have lived,
this is to have succeeded.

RALPH WALDO EMERSON

The secret of happiness is not in doing what one likes, but in liking what one has to do.

JAMES BARRIE

Happiness is an attitude of mind, born of the simple determination to be happy under all outward circumstances. Happiness lies not in things nor in outward attainments. It is the gold of our inner nature, buried beneath the mud of outward sense-cravings.

J. DONALD WALTERS

*If you understand, things are just as
    they are;
If you do not understand, things are just
    as they are.*

Zen koan

A man wandering in the sun retires to the shade of a tree and enjoys the cool atmosphere there. But after a time he is tempted to go out into the hot sun. Again finding the heat unbearable, he returns to the shade. Incessantly he thus moves to and fro, from the shade into the sun and from the sun into the shade. Such a man, we say, is ignorant. A wise man would not quit the shade.

SRI RAMANA MAHARSHI

*You must understand the whole of life,
not just one little part of it. That is why
you must read, that is why you must
look at the skies, that is why you must
sing and dance, and write poems, and
suffer, and understand, for all that
is life.*

J. KRISHNAMURTI

My peace I give unto you: not as the world giveth, give I unto you.

John 14:27

There is no peace except where I am,
    saith the Lord,
I alone remain, I do not change.
As space spreads everywhere and all
    things move and change within it,
But it moves not nor changes,
So I am the space within the soul, of
    which the space without
Is but the similitude or mental image;
Comest thou to inhabit Me thou hast
    the entrance to all life —
Death shall no longer divide thee from
    those thou lovest.
I am the sun that shines upon all
    creatures from within —
Gazest thou upon Me thou shalt be
    filled with joy eternal.
Be not deceived. Soon this outer world
    shall drop off —

Thou shalt slough it away as a man
  sloughs his mortal body.
Learn even now to spread thy wings in
  that other world,
To swim in the ocean, my child, of Me
  and my Love.
Ah, have I not taught thee by the
  semblances of this outer
World, by its alienations and deaths and
  mortal sufferings — all for this,
For joy, ah joy utterable.

EDWARD CARPENTER

Shoot for the moon. Even if you miss it you will land among the stars.

LES BROWN

The miracle is not to fly in the air, or to walk on the water, but to walk on the earth.

Chinese proverb

Let nothing disturb you, let nothing frighten you: everything passes away except God; God alone is sufficient.

ST TERESA OF AVILA

Every blade of grass has its Angel that bends over it and whispers, 'Grow, grow.'

The Talmud

Therefore, unless you make yourself equal to God, you cannot understand God: for the like is not intelligible save to the like. Believe that nothing is impossible for you, thinking yourself immortal and capable of understanding all, all arts, all sciences, the nature of every living being. Mount higher than the highest height, descend lower than the lowest depth. If you embrace in your thought all things at once, times, places, substances, qualities, quantities, you may understand God.

Corpus Hermeticum

Each mortal thing does one thing and
*   the same:*
Deals out that being indoors each one
*   dwells;*
Selves — goes itself; myself it speaks and
*   spells,*
*Crying **What I do is for me: for that***
*   **I came.***

I say more: the just man justices;
Keeps grace: that keeps all his goings
*   graces;*
Acts in God's eye what is God's eye
*   he is —*
Christ.

GERARD MANLEY HOPKINS

Expect your every need to be met,
Expect the answer to every problem,
Expect abundance on every level,
Expect to grow spiritually.

EILEEN CADDY

Ask, and it will be given you.
seek, and you will find;
knock, and it will be opened to you.

Luke 11:9

The Bodhisattva of Compassion
When he meditated deeply
Saw the emptiness of all five skandas
And sundered the bonds that caused
   him suffering.

Hear then!
Form is no other than emptiness
Emptiness no other than form.
Form is only emptiness
Emptiness only form.

Feeling, thought and choice
Consciousness itself
Are the same as this.

All things are the primal void
Which is not born or destroyed
Nor is it stained or pure,
Nor does it wax or wane.

So, in emptiness, no form
No feeling, thought or choice
Nor is there consciousness

No eye, ear, nose, tongue, body, mind;
No colour, sound, smell, taste, touch
Or what the mind takes hold of
Nor even act of sensing.

No ignorance or end of it
Nor all that comes of ignorance;
No withering, no death,
No end of them.

Nor is there pain or cause of pain
Or cease in pain, or noble path
To lead from pain,
Not even wisdom to attain!
Attainment too is emptiness.

So know that the Bodhisattva
Holding to nothing whatever

But dwelling in Prajna wisdom
Is freed of of delusive hindrance
Rid of the fear bred by it
And reaches clearest Nirvana.

All Buddhas of past and present
Buddhas of future time
Using this Prajna wisdom
Come to full and perfect vision.

Hear then the great dharani
The radiant peerless mantra
The Prajnaparamita
Whose words allay all pain;
Hear and believe its truth!

Gate Gate Paragate Parasamgate Bodhi
    Svaha

The Heart Sutra

You may believe that you are responsible
for what you do,
but not for what you think.
The truth is that you are responsible
for what you think,
because it is only at this level that
you can exercise choice.
What you do comes from what you
    think.

A Course in Miracles

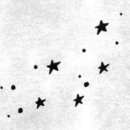

Knowing others is intelligence;
knowing yourself is true wisdom.
Mastering others is strength;
mastering yourself is true power.

LAO-TZU

. . . he allowed himself to be swayed by his conviction that human beings are not born once and for all on the day their mothers give birth to them, but that life obliges them over and over again to give birth to themselves.

GABRIEL GARCIA MARQUEZ

We cannot live only for ourselves. A thousand fibers connect us with our fellow men; and among those fibers, as sympathetic threads, our actions run as causes, and they come back to us as effects.

HERMAN MELVILLE

It is within my power either to serve God, or not to serve Him. Serving Him, I add to my own good and the good of the whole world. Not serving Him, I forfeit my own good and deprive the world of that good, which was in my power to create.

LEO TOLSTOY

We are healed from suffering only by experiencing it to the full.

Suffering only hurts because you fear it. Suffering only hurts because you complain about it. It pursues you only because you flee from it. You must not flee, you must not complain, you must not fear. You must love. You know all this yourself, you know quite well, deep within you, that there is a single magic, a single power, a single salvation, and a single happiness, and that is called loving. Well then, love your suffering. Do not resist it, do not flee from it. Taste how sweet it is in its essence, give yourself to it, do not meet it with aversion. It is only your aversion that hurts, nothing else.

HERMANN HESSE

Everything that happens to you is your teacher. The secret is to learn to sit at the feet of your own life and be taught by it.

Everything that happens is either a blessing which is also a lesson, or a lesson which is also a blessing.

POLLY BERRIEN BERENDS

When the heart weeps for what it has lost, the spirit laughs for what it has found.

Sufi aphorism

Go **with** the pain, let it take you . . .
Open your palms and your body to the
pain. It comes in waves like a tide, and
you must be open as a vessel lying on
the beach, letting it fill you up and
then, retreating, leaving you empty and
clear . . . With a deep breath — it has
to be as deep as the pain — one reaches a
kind of inner freedom from pain, as
though the pain were not yours but your
body's. The spirit lays the body on the
altar.

ANNE MORROW LINDBERGH

*Everything that happens and
everything that befalls us has
    a meaning,
but it is often difficult to recognize it.
Also in the book of life every page
    has two sides:
we human beings fill the upper side
    with our plans, hopes and wishes,
but Providence writes on the other side,
and what it ordains is seldom our goal.*

NISÂMÎ

Let your hook be always cast; in the pool where you least expect it, there will be a fish.

OVID

Each player must accept the cards life deals him or her.

But once they are in hand, he or she alone must decide how to play the cards in order to win the game.

VOLTAIRE

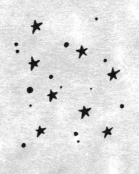

The man with the clear head is the man who . . . looks life in the face, realizes that everything is problematic and feels himself lost . . . Instinctively, as do the shipwrecked, he will look around for something to which to cling, and that tragic, ruthless glance, absolutely sincere, because it is a question of his salvation, will cause him to bring order into the chaos of his life.

JOSÉ ORTEGA Y GASSET

*Rather light a candle than complain
about the darkness.*

We do not see things as they are.
We see them as we are.

The Talmud

Me as I think I am and me as I am in fact — sorrow, in other words, and the ending of sorrow. One third, more or less, of all the sorrow that the person I think I am must endure is unavoidable. It is the sorrow inherent in the human condition, the price we must pay for being sentient and self-conscious organisms, aspirants to liberation, but subject to the laws of nature, and under orders to keep on marching, through irreversible time, through a world that is wholly indifferent to our well-being, towards decrepitude and the certainty of death. The remaining two-thirds of all sorrow is home-made and, so far as the universe is concerned, unnecessary.

ALDOUS HUXLEY

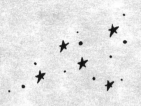

The real voyage of discovery consists not in seeking new landscapes but in having new eyes.

MARCEL PROUST

*You who perceive yourself as weak and
     frail,
with futile hopes and devastated dreams,
born but to die, to weep and suffer pain,
hear this:
All power is given unto you in earth and
     Heaven.
There is nothing that you cannot do.*

A Course in Miracles

You begin to see that there are seasons in your life in the same way as there are seasons in nature. There are times to cultivate and create, when you nurture your world and give birth to new ideas and ventures. There are times of flourishing and abundance, when life feels in full bloom, energized and expanding. And there are times of fruition, when things comes to an end. They have reached their climax and must be harvested before they begin to fade. And finally, of course, there are times that are cold and cutting and empty, times when the spring of new beginnings seems like a distant dream. Those rhythms in life are natural events. They weave into one another as day follows night, bringing, not messages of hope and fear, but messages of how things are. If you realize that each phase of your life is a natural occurrence, then you need not be swayed, pushed up and down by the changes in circumstance and mood that life brings. You find that you have an opportunity to be fully in the world at all times and to show yourself as a brave and proud individual in any circumstance.

CHÖGYAM TRUNGPA

Life is what it is, you cannot change it, but you can change yourself.

HAZRAT INAYAT KHAN

The most powerful thing you can do to change the world, is to change your own beliefs about the nature of life, people, reality to something more positive . . . and begin to act accordingly.

SHAKTI GAWAIN

You shall be free indeed when your days
are not without a care nor your nights
without a want and a grief.

But rather when these things girdle
your life and yet you rise above them
naked and unbound.

KHALIL GIBRAN

If there be righteousness in the heart,
    there will be beauty in the character.
If there be beauty in the character,
    there will be harmony in the home.
If there be harmony in the home,
    there will be order in the nation.
If there be order in the nation,
    there will be peace in the world.

CONFUCIUS

The serious problems in life are never fully solved. If ever they should appear to be so it is a sure sign that something has been lost. The meaning and purpose of a problem seem to lie not in its solution but in our working at it incessantly. This alone preserves us from stultification and petrifaction.

C.G. JUNG

Man is asked to make of himself what he is supposed to become to fulfil his destiny.

PAUL TILLICH

If we could read the secret history of our enemies, we would find in each man's life a sorrow and a suffering enough to disarm all hostility.

HENRY WADSWORTH LONGFELLOW

I was angry with my friend:
I told my wrath, my wrath did end.
I was angry with my foe:
I told it not, my wrath did grow.

WILLIAM BLAKE

The only devils in the world are those running in our own hearts. That is where the battle should be fought.

MAHATMA GANDHI

This above all: to thine own self be true,
And it must follow, as the night the
   day,
Thou canst not then be false to any
   man.

WILLIAM SHAKESPEARE
Hamlet I.iii.

And God shall wipe away all tears from
    their eyes;
and there shall be no more death,
neither sorrow, nor crying, neither shall
there be any more pain: for the former
things are passed away.

Revelation 21:4

Stand through life firm as a rock in the sea, undisturbed and unmoved by its ever-rising waves.

HAZRAT INAYAT KHAN

I who am the beauty of the green earth
    and the white moon among the stars
    and the mysteries of the waters,
I call upon your soul to arise and
    come unto Me.
For I am the soul of nature that
    gives life to the universe.
From Me all things proceed and unto
    Me they must return.
Let My worship be in the heart that
    rejoices, for behold — all acts of love
    and pleasure are My rituals.
Let there be beauty and strength, power
    and compassion, honour and humility,
    mirth and reverence within you.
And you who seek to know Me, know
    that your seeking and yearning will
    avail you not, unless you know the
    Mystery:

*for if that which you seek, you find not
within yourself, you will never find it
    without.
For behold, I have been with you
    from the beginning, and I am that
    which is attained at the end of
    desire.*

TRADITIONAL — *The Charge of the
Goddess — modernized by Starhawk*

The wind blows where it wills, and you hear the sound of it, but you do not know whence it comes or whither it goes; so it is with every one who is born of the Spirit.

John 3:8

From time without beginning, the tree
  of unknowing
Has been watered by the monsoon of
  mental habit.
What a tangle of delusion it has
  become.
Listen. Ponder. Practise.
Chop it down with the axe of the guru's
  instruction.

CAURANGIPA

It is not easy to find happiness in
    ourselves,
and it is not possible to find it elsewhere.

AGNES REPPLIER

Well-being is possible only to the degree to which one has overcome one's narcissism; to the degree to which one is open, responsive, sensitive, awake, empty. Well-being means to be fully related to man and nature affectively, to overcome separateness and alienation, to arrive at the experience of oneness with all that exists . . . Well-being means to be fully born, to become what one potentially is.

ERICH FROMM

The philosophers indeed are clever
    enough, but wanting in wisdom;
As to the others, they are either ignorant
    or puerile!
They take an empty fist as containing
    something real and the pointing
    finger as the object pointed at.
Because the finger is adhered to as
    though it were the Moon, all their
    efforts are lost.

YOKA DAISHI

Your reason and your passion are the rudder and the sails of your seafaring soul.

If either your sails or your rudder be broken, you can but toss and drift, or else be held at a standstill in mid-seas.

For reason, ruling alone, is a force confining; and passion, unattended, is a flame that burns to its own destruction.

Therefore let your soul exalt your reason to the height of passion, that it may sing; And let it direct your passion with reason, that your passion may live through its own daily resurrection, and like the phoenix rise above its own ashes.

KHALIL GIBRAN

The life which is unexamined is not worth living.

PLATO

Suppose a man not blind were to observe the multitudinous bubbles being borne rapidly along on the surface of the river Ganges, and should watch and carefully examine them. After he has carefully examined them they will appear to him empty, unreal and insubstantial. In exactly the same way does the monk behold all corporeal phenomena . . . all feelings . . . all perceptions . . . all mental formations . . . and all states of consciousness, whether they be of the past, the present, or the future . . . far or near. He watches and carefully examines them, and after he has carefully examined them, they appear to him empty, unreal, and insubstantial.

SAMYUTTA-NIKĀYA

*Have you learned lessons only of those
who admired you, and were tender with
you, and stood aside for you? Have you
not learned great lessons from those who
braced themselves against you, and
disputed the passage with you?*

WALT WHITMAN

A clay pot sitting in the sun will always be a clay pot. It has to go through the white heat of the furnace to become porcelain.

MILDRED WITTE STOUVEN

When you get into a tight place and everything goes against you 'til it seems as though you could not hold on a minute longer, never give up then, for that is just the place and time that the tide will turn.

HARRIET BEECHER STOWE

God grant me the serenity to accept the things I cannot change, courage to change the things I can, and wisdom to know the difference.

REINHOLD NIEBUHR

Make your ego porous. Will is of little importance, complaining is nothing, fame is nothing. Openness, patience, receptivity, solitude is everything.

RAINER MARIA RILKE

Some day, after we have mastered the winds, the waves, the tides and gravity, we shall harness . . . the energies of love. Then, for the second time in the history of the world, man will have discovered fire.

TEILHARD DE CHARDIN

The whole world is a market-place of
    Love,
For naught that is, from Love remains
    remote.
The Eternal Wisdom made all things in
    Love:
On Love they all depend, to Love all
    turn.
The earth, the heavens, the sun, the
    moon, the stars
The centre of their orbit find in Love.
By Love are all bewildered, stupefied,
Intoxicated by the Wine of Love.
From each, a mystic silence Love
    demands,
What do all seek so earnestly? 'Tis Love.
Love is the subject of their inmost
    thoughts,
In Love no longer 'Thou' and 'I' exist,

For self has passed away in the Beloved.
Now will I draw aside the veil from
    Love,
And in the temple of mine inmost soul
Behold the Friend, Incomparable Love.
He who would know the secret of both
    worlds
Will find the secret of them both, is
    Love.

'ATTÂR

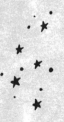

That thou mayest have pleasure in
    everything
     seek pleasure in nothing
That thou mayest know everything
     seek to know nothing
That thou mayest possess all things
     seek to possess nothing
That thou mayest be everything
     seek to be nothing.

ST JOHN OF THE CROSS

Your own body is not your possession . . .
It is the shape lent to you by heaven and
earth. Your life is not your possession; it
is harmony between your forces, granted
for a time by heaven and earth. Your
nature and destiny are not your
possessions; they are the course laid down
for you by heaven and earth. Your
children and grandchildren are not your
possessions; heaven and earth lend them
to you to cast off from your body as an
insect sheds its skin. Therefore you travel
without knowing where you go, stay
without knowing what you cling to, are
fed without knowing how. You are the
breath of heaven and earth which goes to
and fro; how can you ever possess it?

LIEH-TZU

What lies behind us, and what lies before us are tiny matters, compared to what lies within us.

RALPH WALDO EMERSON

Truth is within ourselves, it takes no rise
From outward things, whate'er you may
    believe.
There is an inner centre in us all
Where truth abides in fullness; and
    around
Wall upon wall the gross flesh hems it
    in
That perfect, clear perception which is
    Truth.
A baffling and perverting carnal mesh
Binds all and makes all error, but to
    know
Rather consists in finding out a way
For the imprisoned splendour to escape
Than in achieving entry for a light
Supposed to be without.

ROBERT BROWNING

Truth cannot be framed — it has continually to be discovered. There can only be the truth of the moment, the eternal now. Life in the eternal now is the essential mission.

FRÉDÉRIC LIONEL

If we are truly in the present moment, and not being carried away by our thoughts and fantasies, then we are in a position to be free of fate and available to our destiny. When we are in the present moment, our work on Earth begins.

RESHAD FEILD

It seems to me that one of the greatest stumbling blocks in life is this constant struggle to reach, to achieve, to acquire.

J. KRISHNAMURTI

The greatest griefs are those we cause ourselves.

SOPHOCLES

The quality of mercy is not strained,
It droppeth as the gentle rain from
    heaven
Upon the place beneath: it is twice
    blessed
It blesseth him that gives and him that
    takes.

WILLIAM SHAKESPEARE
The Merchant of Venice IV.i.

. . . something in you dies when you bear the unbearable. And it is only in that dark night of the soul that you are prepared to see as God sees and to love as God loves.

RAM DASS

All that is, at all,
Lasts ever, past recall.
Earth changes, but thy soul and God
* stand sure.*

ROBERT BROWNING

*When one sees Eternity in things that
pass away and Infinity in finite things,
then one has pure knowledge.*

*But if one merely sees the diversity of
things, with their divisions and
limitations, then one has impure
knowledge.*

*And if one selfishly sees a thing as if it
were everything, independent of the
ONE and the many, then one is in the
darkness of ignorance.*

Bhagavad Gita

The secret of life is balance, and the absence of balance is life's destruction.

HAZRAT INAYAT KHAN

I was as sure as that I was alive, that happiness not only needs no justification, but that it is also the only final test of whether what I am doing is right for me. Only of course happiness is not the same as pleasure; it includes the pain of losing as well as the pleasure of finding.

JOANNA FIELD

Go placidly amid the noise and the haste, and remember what peace there may be in silence.

As far as possible, without surrender, be on good terms with all persons.

Speak your truth quietly and clearly; and listen to others, even to the dull and the ignorant; they too have their story.

Avoid loud and aggressive persons; they are vexatious to the spirit.

If you compare yourself with others, you may become vain or bitter, for always there will be greater and lesser persons than yourself.

Enjoy your achievements as well as your plans.

Keep interested in your own career, however humble; it is a real possession in the changing fortunes of time.

Exercise caution in your business affairs, for the world is full of trickery. But let this not blind you to what virtue there is; many persons strive for high ideals, and everywhere life is full of heroism.

Be yourself. Especially do not feign affection.

Neither be cynical about love; for in the face of all aridity and disenchantment it is as perennial as the grass.

Take kindly the counsel of the years, gracefully surrendering the things of youth.

Nurture strength of spirit to shield you in sudden misfortune.

But do not distress yourself with dark imaginings. Many fears are born of fatigue and loneliness.

Beyond a wholesome discipline, be gentle with yourself.

You are a child of the universe no less than the trees and the stars; you have a right to be here.

And whether or not it is clear to you, no doubt the universe is unfolding as it should.

Therefore be at peace with God, whatever you conceive Him to be.

And whatever your labors and aspirations, in the noisy confusion of life, keep peace in your soul.

With all its sham, drudgery and broken dreams, it is still a beautiful world.

Be cheerful. Strive to be happy.

MAX EHRMANN

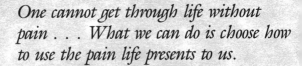

One cannot get through life without pain . . . What we can do is choose how to use the pain life presents to us.

BERNIE S. SIEGEL

*The mark of your ignorance is the depth
of your belief in injustice and tragedy.
    What the caterpillar calls the end of
the world, the master calls a butterfly.*

RICHARD BACH

We live on the brink of disaster because we do not know how to let life alone. We do not respect the living and fruitful contradictions and paradoxes of which true life is full.

THOMAS MERTON

Turn your face to the sun and the shadows fall behind you.

Maori proverb

Vex not thy spirit at the course of things; they heed not thy vexation. How ludicrous and outlandish is astonishment at anything that may happen in life.

MARCUS AURELIUS

Instead of seeing the rug being pulled from under us, we can learn to dance on a shifting carpet.

THOMAS CRUM

I will lift up mine eyes unto the hills,
   from whence cometh my help.
My help cometh from the Lord, which
   made heaven and earth.
He will not suffer thy foot to be moved:
   he that keepeth thee will not slumber.
Behold he that keepeth Israel shall
   neither slumber nor sleep.
The Lord is thy keeper: the Lord is thy
   shade upon thy right hand.
The sun shall not smite thee by day, nor
   the moon by night.
The Lord shall preserve thee from all
   evil: he shall preserve thy soul.
The Lord shall preserve thy going out
   and thy coming in from this time
   forth, and even for evermore.

Psalm 121

The winds of grace blow all the time.
All we need to do is set our sails.

RAMAKRISHNA

Our life is what our thoughts make of it.

MARCUS AURELIUS

All that we are is the result of what we have thought: all that we are is founded on our thoughts and formed of our thoughts. If a man speaks or acts with an evil thought, pain pursues him, as the wheel of the wagon follows the hoof of the ox that draws it.

All that we are is the result of what we have thought: all that we are is founded on our thoughts and formed of our thoughts. If a man speaks or acts with a pure thought, happiness pursues him like his own shadow that never leaves him.

The Dhammapada

A worldly loss often turns into spiritual gain.

HAZRAT INAYAT KHAN

How else but through a broken heart
May Lord Christ enter in.

OSCAR WILDE
The Ballad of Reading Gaol

To every disadvantage there is a corresponding advantage.

W. CLEMENT STONE

To improve the golden moment of opportunity, and catch the good that is within our reach, is the great art of life.

WILLIAM JAMES

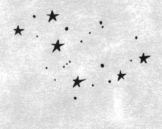

*You cannot stay on the summit forever;
you have to come down again . . . So
why bother in the first place? Just this:
what is above knows what is below, but
what is below does not know what is
above.*

RENÉ DAUMAL

No man is an island, entire of itself;
every man is a piece of the continent, a
part of the main. If a clod be washed
away by the sea, Europe is the less, as
well as if a promontory were, as well as if
a manor of thy friend's or of thy own
were. Any man's death diminishes me
because I am involved in mankind, and
therefore never send to know for whom
the bell tolls, it tolls for thee.

JOHN DONNE

From Unreality, lead me to Reality,
From Darkness, lead me unto Light,
From Death, lead me to Immortality.

The Upanishads

*Our hearts are restless until they find
their rest in thee.*

ST AUGUSTINE

Breathe through the hearts of our desire
Thy coolness and thy balm;
Let sense be dumb, Let flesh retire;
Breath through the earthquake, wind,
    and fire
O still small voice of calm!

JOHN WHITTIER

Love becomes the ultimate answer to the ultimate human question.

ARCHIBALD MACLEISH

What could you want
forgiveness cannot give?
Do you want peace? Forgiveness offers it.
Do you want happiness, a quiet mind,
a certainty of purpose,
and a sense of worth and beauty
that transcends the world?
Do you want care and safety,
and the warmth of sure protection
      always?
Do you want a quietness that cannot be
      disturbed,
a gentleness that never can be hurt,
a deep, abiding comfort,
and a rest so perfect it can never be
      upset?
All this forgiveness offers you.

A Course in Miracles

My religion is very simple — my religion is kindness.

DALAI LAMA

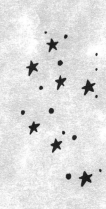

The greatest discovery of my generation is that human beings can alter their lives by altering their attitudes of mind.

WILLIAM JAMES

*Each man is his own absolute law-giver,
the dispenser of glory or gloom to himself;
the decreer of his life, his reward, his
punishment.*

MABEL COLLINS

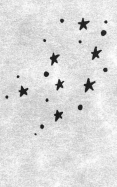

Life does not consist mainly — or even largely — of facts and happenings. It consists mainly of the storm of thoughts that are forever blowing through one's mind.

MARK TWAIN

I will greet this day with love in my heart. And how will I do this? Henceforth will I look on all things with love and I will be born again. I will love the sun for it warms my bones; yet I will love the rain for it cleanses my spirit. I will love the light for it shows me the way; yet I will love the darkness for it shows me the stars. I will welcome happiness for it enlarges my heart; yet I will endure sadness for it opens my soul. I will acknowledge rewards for they are my due; yet I will welcome obstacles for they are my challenge.

OG MANDINO

Said one oyster to a neighbouring oyster, 'I have a very great pain within me. It is heavy and round and I am in distress.'

And the other oyster replied with haughty complacence, 'Praise be to the heavens and to the sea, I have no pain within me. I am well and whole both within and without.'

At that moment a crab was passing by and heard the two oysters, and he said to the one who was well and whole both within and without, 'Yes, you are well and whole; but the pain that your neighbour bears is a pearl of exceeding beauty.'

KHALIL GIBRAN

It may be that some little root of the sacred tree still lives. Nourish it then, that it may leaf and bloom and fill with singing birds.

BLACK ELK

When a man finds that it is his destiny to suffer, he will have to accept his suffering as his task; his single and unique task. He will have to acknowledge the fact that even in suffering he is unique and alone in the universe. No one can relieve him of his suffering or suffer in his place. His unique opportunity lies in the way in which he bears his burden.

VIKTOR FRANKL

Life is difficult.

This is a great truth, one of the greatest truths. It is a great truth because once we truly see this truth, we transcend it. Once we truly know that life is difficult — once we truly understand and accept it — then life is no longer difficult. Because once it is accepted, the fact that life is difficult no longer matters.

M. SCOTT PECK

I will call the **world** a School instituted
for the purpose of teaching little children
to read — I will call the **human heart**
the **horn book** used in that school and I
will call the **Child able to read,** the
Soul made from that **school** and its
horn book. Do you not see how necessary
a World of Pains and troubles is to
school an Intelligence and make it a
Soul? A Place where the heart must feel
and suffer in a thousand diverse ways!
Not merely is the Heart a Hornbook,
it is the Mind's Bible, it is the Mind's
experience, it is the test from which
the Mind or intelligence sucks its
identity . . . And what are proovings of
[man's] heart but fortifiers or alterers of
his nature? And what is his altered
nature but his Soul? — and what was

his Soul before it came into the world and had these proovings and alterations and perfectionings? An intelligence — without Identity — and how is this Identity to be made? Through the medium of the Heart? And how is the heart to become this Medium but in a world of Circumstances.

JOHN KEATS

Your pain is the breaking of the shell that encloses your understanding.

Even as the stone of the fruit must break, that its heart may stand in the sun, so must you know pain.

And could you keep your heart in wonder at the daily miracles of your life, your pain would not seem less wondrous than your joy;

And you would accept the seasons of your heart, even as you have always accepted the seasons that pass over your fields.

And you would watch with serenity through the winters of your grief.

Much of your pain is self-chosen.

It is the bitter potion by which the physician within you heals your sick self.

Therefore trust the physician, and drink his remedy in silence and tranquillity:

For his hand, though heavy and hard, is guided by the tender hand of the Unseen,

And the cup he brings, though it burn your lips, has been fashioned of the clay which the

Potter has moistened with His own sacred tears.

KHALIL GIBRAN

*Death and transformation are man's
unchosen and unchangeable fate. All
that he can choose and change is
consciousness. But to change this is to
change all.*

RODNEY COLLIN

In times of suffering, when you feel abandoned, perhaps even annihilated, there is occurring — at levels deeper than your pain — the entry of the sacred, the possibility of redemption. Wounding opens the doors of our sensibility to a larger reality . . . Pathos gives us eyes and ears to see and hear what our normal eyes and ears cannot.

JEAN HOUSTON

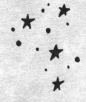

Never measure the height of a mountain, until you have reached the top. Then you will see how low it was.

DAG HAMMARSKJÖLD

*Let him who seeks not cease from seeking
until he finds;
and when he finds,
he will be disturbed;
and when he is disturbed,
he will marvel,
and he shall reign over the All.*

The Gospel of Thomas

*If the doors of perception were cleansed
everything would appear to man as it is,
infinite.*

WILLIAM BLAKE

To him that overcometh will I give to eat
of the tree of life, which is in the midst
of the paradise of God.

Revelation 2:7

What after all, did the king do? He watched his conduct carefully and turned his face southward solemnly. Nothing more.

CONFUCIUS

It is a rare life that remains well ordered even in private. Any man can play his part in the side show and represent a worthy man on the boards; but to be disciplined within, in his own bosom, where all is permissible, where all is concealed — that's the point.

MICHEL DE MONTAIGNE

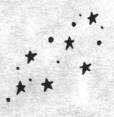

The individual moves towards BEING, knowingly and acceptingly, the process he inwardly and actually is. He moves away from being what he is not, from being a facade. He is not trying to be more than he is, with the attendant feelings of guilt or self-depreciation. He is increasingly listening to the deepest recesses of his physiological and emotional being, and finds himself increasingly willing to be, with greater accuracy and depth, that self which he most truly is.

CARL ROGERS

Whither shall I go from thy spirit? or
whither shall I flee from thy
presence?
If I ascend up into heaven, thou art
there: if I make my bed in hell, thou
art there.
If I take the wings of the morning, and
dwell in the uttermost parts of the
sea;
Even there shall thy hand lead me, and
thy right hand shall hold me.

Psalm 139:7–10

The stream of creation and dissolution never stops . . . All things come out of the one, and the one out of all things.

HERACLITUS

In ascent or descent there is no fixed rule, except that one must do nothing evil. In advance or retreat no sustained perseverance avails, except that one must not depart from one's nature. The superior man fosters his character and labours at his task in order to do everything at the right time. Therefore he makes no mistake.

CONFUCIUS

Love is not getting, but giving. It is sacrifice. And sacrifice is glorious!

JOANNA FIELD

*One finds love not by **being** loved, but by loving.*

We can never know love if we try to draw others to ourselves; nor can we find it by centering our love in them. For love is infinite; it is never ours to create. We can only channel it from its source in Infinity to all whom we meet.

J. DONALD WALTERS

To every thing there is a season, and a time to every purpose under the heaven;

A time to be born, and a time to die; a time to plant, and a time to pluck up that which is planted;

A time to kill, and a time to heal; a time to break down, and a time to build up;

A time to weep, and a time to laugh; a time to mourn, and a time to dance;

A time to cast away stones, and a time to gather stones together; a time to embrace, and a time to refrain from embracing;

A time to get, and a time to lose; a time to keep, and a time to cast away;

A time to rend, and a time to sew, a time to keep silence, and a time to speak;

A time to love, and a time to hate; a time of war, and a time of peace.

Ecclesiastes 3:1–8

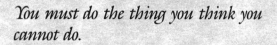

You must do the thing you think you cannot do.

ELEANOR ROOSEVELT

All we are asked to bear we can bear.
That is a law of the spiritual life. The
only hindrance to the working of this
law, as of all benign laws, is fear.

ELIZABETH GOUDGE

The weariest night, the longest day, sooner or later must perforce come to an end.

BARONESS ORCZY

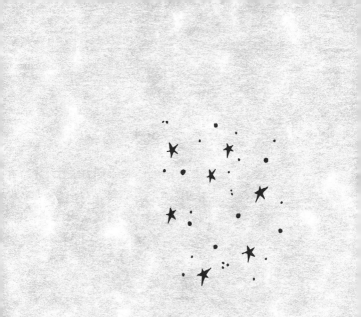

Ye shall know the truth and the truth shall make you free.

John 8:32

*They said to Him: Shall we then, being children, enter the Kingdom? Jesus said to them: When you make the two one, and when you make the inner as the outer and the outer as the inner and the above as the below, and when
you make the male and the female into
a single one,
then you shall enter the Kingdom.*

The Gospel of St Thomas

You who want peace
can find it only by complete forgiveness.

A Course in Miracles

*Needs can be fulfilled, but desires
    cannot be.
Desire is a need gone mad.
Needs are simple, they come from
    nature;
Desires are very complex, they don't come
    from nature.
They are created by the mind.
Needs are moment to moment,
    they are created out of life itself,
Desires are not moment to moment,
    they are always for the future.
They are not created by life itself,
    they are projected by the mind.*

BHAGWAN SHREE RAJNEESH

One is happy as a result of one's own efforts, once one knows the necessary ingredients of happiness — simple tastes, a certain degree of courage, self-denial to a point, love of work, and above all, a clear conscience. Happiness is no vague dream, of that I now feel certain.

GEORGE SAND

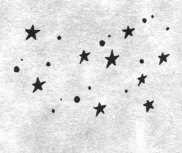

. . . we could never learn to be brave and patient if there were only joy in the world.

HELEN KELLER

The individual who withdraws his shadow from his neighbour and finds it in himself and is reconciled to it as to an estranged brother is doing a task of great universal importance.

LAURENS VAN DER POST

Insomuch as love grows in you so in you beauty grows. For love is the beauty of the soul.

ST AUGUSTINE

*Happy is the man that findeth wisdom,
and the man that getteth
understanding.*

*For the gaining of it is better than the
gaining of silver, and the profit thereof
than fine gold.*

She is more precious than rubies:

*And none of the things thou canst desire
are to be compared with her . . .*

*Her ways are ways of pleasantness,
and all her paths are peace.*

Proverbs 3:13–17

Come to the edge
He said. They said:
We are afraid.
Come to the edge
He said. They came.
He pushed them, and
they flew . . .

GUILLAUME APOLLINAIRE

There is only one courage and that is the courage to go on dying to the past, not to collect it, not to accumulate it, not to cling to it. We all cling to the past, and because we cling to the past we become unavailable to the present.

BHAGWAN SHREE RAJNEESH

Ask, and it shall be given you; seek, and ye shall find; knock, and it shall be opened unto you: For everyone that asketh receiveth; and he that seeketh findeth; and to him that knocketh it shall be opened.

Matthew 7:7–8

All creatures . . . are the same life, the same essence, the same power, the same one and nothing less.

HENRY SUSO

From the point of Light
    within the Mind of God
Let the light stream forth into
    the minds of men.
Let Light descend on Earth.

From the point of Love
    within the Heart of God
Let love stream forth into
    the hearts of men.
May Christ return to Earth.

From the centre where the
    Will of God is known
Let purpose guide the little
    wills of men —
The purpose which The
    Masters know and serve.

From the centre which we
    call the race of man
Let the Plan of Love and
    Light work out
And may it seal the door
    where evil dwells.

Let Light and Love and
    Power restore the Plan
    on Earth.

ALICE BAILEY

What is within us is also without.
What is without us is also within.

The Upanishads

No man can reveal to you aught but
    that which already lies half asleep in
    the dawning of your knowledge.

The teacher who walks in the shadow of
    the temple, among his followers, gives
    not of his wisdom but rather of
    his faith and his lovingness.

If he is indeed wise he does not bid
    you enter the house of his wisdom,
    but rather leads you to the threshold
    of your own mind.

KHALIL GIBRAN

Two birds
    inseparable companions
    perch on the same tree.
One eats the fruit,
    the other looks on.

The first bird is our individual self,
    feeding on the pleasures and pains of
    this world;
The other is the universal Self,
    silently witnessing all.

Mundaya Upanishad

The greatest human quest is to know what one must do in order to become a human being.

IMMANUEL KANT

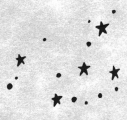

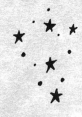

If God is anything, he is understanding . . .

Understanding is acquired by means of suffering or distress or experience.

Will, desire, pain, envy etc. are all natural. But understanding is acquired.

WILLIAM BLAKE

Every new born being indeed comes fresh and blithe into the new existence, and enjoys it as a free gift: but there is, and can be, nothing freely given. Its fresh existence is paid for by the old age and death of a worn-out existence which has perished, but which contained the indestructible seed out of which this new existence has arisen: they are one being.

ARTHUR SCHOPENHAUER

Everything is so dangerous that nothing is really very frightening.

GERTRUDE STEIN

*All shall be well, and all shall be well
and all manner of things shall be well.*

JULIAN OF NORWICH

All nature is but art unknown to thee;
All chance, direction which thou canst
not see.

ALEXANDER POPE

Nothing we ever imagined is beyond our powers, only beyond our present self-knowledge.

THEODORE ROSZAK

Are you in earnest? Then seize
this very minute.
What you can do, or dream you can,
    begin it;
Boldness has genius, power and magic in
    it;
only engage and then the mind
    grows heated;
Begin, and then the work will be
    completed.

J.W. VON GOETHE

Where shall we begin?

There is no beginning. Start where you arrive. Stop before what entices you. And work! You will enter little by little into the entirety. Method will be born in proportion to your interest . . .

In the calm exile of work, we must learn patience, which in turn teaches energy, and energy gives us eternal youth made of self-collectedness and enthusiasm.

ANGUSTE RODIN

I do my thing, and you do your thing,
I am not in this world to live up to your expectations
And you are not in this world to live up to mine.
You are you and I am I,
And if by chance we find each other, it's beautiful.
If not, it can't be helped.

FREDERICK S. PERLS

. . . *You don't get to choose how you're going to die. Or when. You can only decide how you're going to live. Now.*

JOAN BAEZ

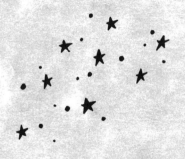

To keep a lamp burning we have to keep putting oil in it.

MOTHER TERESA

Love is the law of God. You live that you may learn to love. You love that you may learn to live. No other lesson is required of man.

MIKHAIL NAIMY

The Japanese master Nan-in gave
    audience
to a professor of philosophy.
Serving tea, Nan-in filled his visitor's
    cup,
and kept pouring.

The professor watched the overflow
until he could restrain himself no
    longer:
Stop!
The cup is overfull, no more will go in.

Nan-in said:
Like this cup,
you are full of your own opinions and
    speculations.
How can I show you Zen
unless you first empty your cup?

Zen story

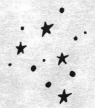

*Strong in their softness are the sprays of
    the wisteria creeper;
The pine in its hardness is broken by the
    weak snow.*

MASTER JUKYU

Those whose lives are fruitful to themselves, to their friends or to the world are inspired by hope and sustained by joy; they see in imagination the things that might be and the way in which they are to be brought into existence. In their private relations they are not preoccupied with anxiety lest they should lose such affection and respect as they receive; they are engaged in giving affection and respect, freely, and the reward comes of itself without their seeking. In their work they are not haunted by jealousy of competitors, but are concerned with the actual matter that has to be done. In politics they do not spend time and passion defending unjust privileges of their clan or nation, but they aim at making the world as a whole happier, less cruel, less full of conflict between rival creeds and more full of human beings whose growth has not been dwarfed and stunted by oppression.

BERTRAND RUSSELL

*We learn wisdom from failure much
more than from success; we often discover
what will do, by finding out what will
not do; and probably he who never made
a mistake never made a discovery.*

SAMUEL SMILES

It is in self-limitation that a master first shows himself.

J.W. VON GOETHE

If one advances confidently in the direction of his dreams, and endeavours to live the life which he has imagined, he will meet with a success unexpected in common hours.

HENRY DAVID THOREAU

If we stand tall it is because we stand on the shoulders of many ancestors.

Yoruba proverb

. . . I refuse to be intimidated by
  reality anymore.
After all, what is reality anyway?
  Nothin' but a collective hunch . . .
I made some studies, and
reality is the leading cause of stress
  amongst those in
touch with it. I can take it in small
  doses, but as a lifestyle
I found it too confining.

JANE WAGNER

Nature attains perfection, but a man never does. There is a perfect ant, a perfect bee, but man is perpetually unfinished. He is both an unfinished animal and an unfinished man. It is this incurable unfinishedness which sets man apart from other living things for, in the attempt to finish himself, man becomes a creator. Moreover, the incurable unfinishedness keeps man perpetually immature, perpetually capable of learning and growth.

ERIC HOFFER

I seek the truth everywhere, and respect it wherever I find it, and I submit to it whenever it is shown to me.

FREDERICK THE GREAT

Lord, make me an instrument of thy
    peace.
Where there is hatred, let me sow love;
Where there is injury, pardon;
Where there is doubt, faith;
Where there is despair, hope;
Where there is darkness, light;
Where there is sadness, joy.

O Divine Master, grant that I may not
    so much seek
To be consoled as to console
To be understood as to understand,
To be loved as to love;
For it is in giving that we receive;
It is in pardoning that we are pardoned;
It is in dying that we are born to
    eternal life.

ST FRANCIS OF ASSISI

We shall never cease from exploration
And the end of all our exploring
Will be to arrive where we started
And know the place for the first time.

T.S. ELIOT
Little Gidding

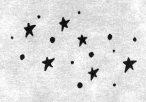

Acknowledgements

The editor would like to thank the following authors and publishers for permission to reprint material from their books:

Caddy, Eileen, *Footprints on the Path*, © 1976 Eileen Caddy, and *The Dawn of Change*, © 1979 Findhorn Foundation. Published by Findhorn Press, The Park, Findhorn, Forres IV36 0TZ, Scotland.

Eliot, T.S., 'Little Gidding' from *Four Quartets*, © 1979 The Estate of T.S. Eliot.

Gibran, Khalil, *The Prophet*, © 1923 Khalil Gibran, renewal © 1951 Administrators CTA. Published by Knopf New York, 1961.

Khan, Hazrat Inayat, *Gayan Vadan Nirtan*, © 1980 Sufi Order. Sufi Order Publications, Lebanon Springs, New York.

Lao Tzu, *Tao Te Ching*, tr. Stephen Mitchell © 1988. Published by Macmillan, 1989.

Mandino, Og, *The Greatest Salesman in the World*. Frederick Fell, Hollywood, Florida, 1968.

Rodegast, Pat and Stanton, Judith, *Emmanuel's Book: A Manual for living comfortably in the cosmos*, © 1985 Pat Rodegast. A Bantam Book published by arrangement with Friends' Press.

Vaughan, Frances and Walsh, Roger (eds.) *Accept This Gift: Selections from A Course in Miracles*, © Foundation for Inner Peace. Published by Jeremy Tarcher, Los Angeles, 1983, and *A Gift of Peace: Selections From A Course in Miracles*, © Foundation for Inner Peace. Published by Jeremy Tarcher, Los Angeles, 1986.

Walters, J. Donald, *Affirmations and Prayers*, © 1988 J. Donald Walters. Crystal Clarity Publishers, Nevada City, California.

Recommended Reading

Bach, Richard, *Illusions* (Pan Books, London, 1979).

Berends, Polly Berrien, *Coming to Life: Travelling the spiritual path in everyday life* (Harper San Francisco, 1990).

Collins, Mabel, *Light on the Path/ Through the Gates of Gold* (Theosophical University Press, Pasadena, California, 1971).

Emerson, Ralph Waldo (ed.), *Works of Ralph Waldo Emerson*, with an introduction by J.P. (Nimmo, Hay & Mitchell, Edinburgh, 1906).

Fromm, Erich, *The Art of Loving* (Allen & Unwin, London, 1957).

Gawain, Shatki, *Creative Visualization* (Whatever Publishing, Mill Valley, California, 1978).

Godwin, Joscelyn (ed.), *Paul Brunton Essential Readings* (The Aquarian Press, London, 1990).

Graham, A.C., *The Book of Lieh-Tzu* (Mandala, London, 1991).

Hayward, Susan, *A Guide for the Advanced Soul: A book of insight* (In-Tune Books, NSW, Australia, 1985).

—, *Begin It Now: A book of motivation* (In-Tune Books , NSW, Australia, 1987).

Houston, Jean, *Search for the Beloved* (The Aquarian Press, London, 1990).

Huxley, Aldous, *The Perennial Philosophy* (Fontana, London, 1958).

Jung, C.G., *Memories, Dreams, Reflections* (Fontana, London, 1972).

—, *Collected Works* (Routledge, London, and Princeton University Press, New Jersey, 1978-90).

Nair, Keshavan, *Beyond Winning* (Paradox Press, Pheonix, Arizona, 1988).

Peck, M. Scott, *The Road Less Travelled: A new psychology of love, traditional values and spiritual growth* (Hutchinson, London, 1983).

Rajneesh, Bhagwan Shree, *Roots and Wings: Talks on Zen* © 1975 Rajneesh Foundation, Poona, India. (First published in India, 1975; published RKP, London, Boston and Henley, 1979).

Safransky, Sy (ed.), *Sunbeams: A Book of Quotations* (North Atlantic Books, Berkeley, California, 1990).

Sangharakshita, *A Survey of Buddhism* (Shambhala, Boulder, 1980).

Siegel, Bernie S., *Love, Medicine and Miracles: Lessons learned about self-healing from a surgeon's experience* (Harper and Row, New York, 1986).

Starhawk, *The Spiral Dance: A rebirth of the ancient religion of the Great Goddess* (Harper San Francisco, 1979).

Trevelyan, George, *Magic Casements: The use of poetry in the expanding of consciousness* (Coventure, London, 1980).

Trine, Ralph Waldo, *In Tune with the Infinite* (G. Bell, London, 1930).

Trungpa, Chögyam, *The Myth of Freedom and the Way of Meditation* (Shambhala, Boulder, 1976).

—, *Cutting through Spiritual Materialism* (Shambhala, Boulder, 1973).

Wagner, Jane, *The Search for Signs of Intelligent Life in the Universe* (Harper and Row, New York, 1986).

Yogananda, Paramahansa, *Autobiography of a Yogi* (Rider, London, 1969).